Obs and Gynae

PG Focus Series

Gestational Diabetes Mellitus

Obs and Gynae
PG Focus Series
Gestational Diabetes Mellitus

Editors

Komal N Chavan
MD DNB MNAMS FCPS DGO FICOG and Diploma in Reproductive Medicine (UK-SH Germany)
Senior Consultant and Unit Chief
Department of Obstetrics and Gynaecology
VN Desai Hospital
Mumbai, Maharashtra, India

Niranjan Chavan
MD FICOG FCPS DGO DFP MICOG DICOG Diploma in Endoscopy (USA)
Professor and Unit Chief
Department of Obstetrics and Gynaecology
Lokmanya Tilak Medical College and General Hospital
Mumbai, Maharashtra, India

Co-Editors

Smurti Kamble
MBBS MS (Obs/Gynae) FMAS
Advanced Diploma in ART and Reproductive Medicine, Kiel
Assistant Professor
Department of Obstetrics and Gynaecology
Lokmanya Tilak Medical College and General Hospital
Mumbai, Maharashtra, India

Swara Patel
MBBS MS DNB (Obs/Gynae)
Assistant Professor
Department of Obstetrics and Gynaecology
Lokmanya Tilak Medical College and General Hospital
Mumbai, Maharashtra, India

JAYPEE BROTHERS MEDICAL PUBLISHERS
The Health Sciences Publisher
New Delhi | London

Jaypee Brothers Medical Publishers (P) Ltd

Headquarters
Jaypee Brothers Medical Publishers (P) Ltd
EMCA House, 23/23-B
Ansari Road, Daryaganj
New Delhi 110 002, India
Landline: +91-11-23272143, +91-11-23272703
+91-11-23282021, +91-11-23245672
Email: jaypee@jaypeebrothers.com

Corporate Office
Jaypee Brothers Medical Publishers (P) Ltd
4838/24, Ansari Road, Daryaganj
New Delhi 110 002, India
Phone: +91-11-43574357
Fax: +91-11-43574314
Email: jaypee@jaypeebrothers.com

Overseas Office
JP Medical Ltd.
83, Victoria Street, London
SW1H 0HW (UK)
Phone: +44 20 3170 8910
Fax: +44 (0)20 3008 6180
Email: info@jpmedpub.com

Website: www.jaypeebrothers.com
Website: www.jaypeedigital.com

Inquiries for bulk sales may be solicited at: jaypee@jaypeebrothers.com

Obs and Gynae PG Focus Series: Gestational Diabetes Mellitus

First Edition: **2025**

ISBN: 978-93-6616-152-5

Printed in India

Preface

Diabetes in pregnancy is a critical and growing concern in modern obstetrics, with significant implications for both maternal and fetal health. As the prevalence of diabetes continues to rise globally, understanding and managing diabetes during pregnancy has become a cornerstone of antenatal care. Whether it is pre-existing type 1 or type 2 diabetes, or gestational diabetes that develops during pregnancy, effective management is essential to minimize complications and ensure the well-being of both mother and baby.

This book aims to provide an in-depth, evidence-based resource for students looking to understand the complexities of diabetes as well as practitioners who are involved in the care of pregnant women with diabetes. It explains in simple language the pathophysiology, diagnosis, and management strategies for diabetes during pregnancy. It also addresses the long-term implications for both maternal health and offspring, as well as the evolving research that shapes current best practices.

We have strived to make every chapter comprehensive with the latest guidelines while also covering practical guidance on managing common challenges, such as optimizing glycemic control, preventing complications like preeclampsia and fetal macrosomia, and coordinating care in multidisciplinary settings.

As our understanding of diabetes in pregnancy continues to evolve, this book aims to remain a valuable resource in navigating the complexities of this condition, and in empowering clinicians to deliver the highest standard of care.

Editors
Komal N Chavan
Niranjan Chavan

Co-Editors
Smurti Kamble
Swara Patel

Acknowledgments

We express our gratitude to all those who contributed to the completion of this book on *Gestational Diabetes Mellitus*. This endeavor would not have been possible without the constant support of many individuals.

We are thankful to all the authors and co-authors for sharing their expertise and commitment to producing a resource of the highest standards.

We are grateful to our mentors and colleagues, whose valuable guidance helped us form the structure and contents of this book.

Our deepest gratitude to our families and friends for their unwavering support, patience, and encouragement during the demanding phases of this project have been our greatest strength.

We are extremely thankful to the President of FOGSI, Dr Jaydeep Tank for supporting this project.

We acknowledge the support of Shri Jitendar P Vij (Group Chairman) and Mr Ankit Vij (Managing Director) of M/s Jaypee Brothers Medical Publishers (P) Ltd, New Delhi, India, in publishing the book and their associates, particularly Ms Chetna Malhotra (Senior Director—Professional Publishing, Marketing, and Business Development), Ms Kritika Dua (Senior Commissioning Editor), and Ms Pragati Singh (Development Editor), who have been prompt, efficient, and most helpful.

Lastly, we hope that the postgraduate students find this book useful in their examinations and teachers for a quick revision. We also hope this book serves as a valuable resource, contributing to the betterment of patient care and surgical practice to the practicing obstetricians and gynaecologists.

Thank you all for being a part of this journey.

Contents

CHAPTER 1

Introduction

In the era of newly emerging infectious pandemics, diabetes remains the endocrinologic pandemic owing to a sedentary lifestyle, lack of activity, and unhealthy eating habits. Pregnancy being a diabetogenic state subjects a large proportion of the population to adverse maternal and perinatal morbidity. The International Association of Diabetes and Pregnancy Study Groups (IADPSG) and the World Health Organization (WHO) have classified hyperglycemia in pregnancy (HIP) into three categories:

1. Pregestational diabetes
2. Overt diabetes in pregnancy (DIP)
3. Gestational diabetes mellitus (GDM)

Gestational diabetes mellitus is currently defined as any degree of glucose intolerance with onset or first recognition during pregnancy.

Gestational diabetes mellitus arises due to insulin resistance that develops during pregnancy secondary to the action of pregnancy-specific hormones. Clinically GDM ranges from asymptomatic to severe hyperglycemia and its complications. GDM is associated with an increased risk of short-term as well as long-term adverse effects for both mother and baby and hence its diagnosis and adequate treatment are of prime importance. Women with GDM are at an increased risk of developing type 2 diabetes mellitus (DM) 5–6 years after pregnancy while babies born to such mothers have the risk of becoming obese in their adulthood with further risk of development of type 2 DM.

HISTORY

The history of diabetes mellitus dates back to 1500 BC. when it was described in the Egyptian Ebers Papyrus.[1] In 1824 Bennewitz in Germany described the first clinical case of a woman with intensive thirst and recurrent glycosuria in three successive pregnancies. One of her babies weighed almost 5.5 kg and her urine contained a big amount of saccharine matter.[2] In 1945, Miller reported the first observations of obstetrical complications in the prediabetic period.[3] In the 1950s the risk factors for the development of abnormalities in carbohydrate metabolism in pregnancy were defined and the term GDM became accepted. Being overweight, obese, and of non-European ethnicity along with a history of GDM in a previous pregnancy, history of diabetes, previous stillbirth, macrosomia, and polycystic ovarian syndrome are major risk factors for HIP.

EPIDEMIOLOGY

Presently, the International Diabetes Federation 2019 estimates 20.4 million global live births (15.8%) to women with HIP.[4] Pregestational diabetes affects 1–5% of people worldwide and has been on the rise in women aged >40 years. Owing to the lower standard fertility ratio in women with type 1 diabetes, the prevalence of type 1 diabetes in nonpregnant women is more than that in pregnancy. Type 1 DM complicates about 0.3–0.8% of pregnancies; type 2 DM affects the remaining patients, and a tiny percentage has uncommon forms of the disease. DIP is prevalent in 0.2–4% of cases, primarily postpartum type 2 DM.

INDIAN PERSPECTIVE

There is wide variability in the reported prevalence rate for GDM in India, varying from <4% to nearly 18%. The overall prevalence is approximately 7%, higher in urban versus rural areas, among older age groups, and higher socioeconomic status (SES) groups.[5] The prevalence of gestational diabetes has been reported to range from 3.8% in Kashmir to 6.2% in Mysore, 9.5% in Western India, and 17.9% in Tamil Nadu.[6] The wide variation of prevalence in India can be attributed to the wide differences in the dietary habits, living conditions, and socioeconomic levels of the population in different states of the country. The incidence of GDM is expected to increase to 20%, i.e., one in every five pregnant women is likely to have GDM.

The increasing prevalence of HIP has a significant impact on public health expenditure required for both diagnosis and management of the disease and its complications.

REFERENCES

1. Karamanou M, Protogerou A, Tsoucalas G, Androutsos G, Poulakou-Rebelakou E. Milestones in the history of diabetes mellitus: The main contributors. World J Diabetes. 2016;7(1):1-7.
2. Hadden DR, Hillebrand B. The first recorded case of diabetic pregnancy (Bennewitz HG, 1824, University of Berlin). Diabetologia. 1989;32(8):625.
3. Miller HC. The effect of the prediabetic state on the survival of the fetus and the birth weight of the newborn infant. N Engl J Med. 1945;233:376-8.
4. International Diabetes Federation. IDF Diabetes Atlas, 9th edition. Belgium: International Diabetes Federation; 2019. p. 168.
5. Swaminathan G, Swaminathan A, Corsi DJ. Prevalence of Gestational Diabetes in India by Individual Socioeconomic, Demographic, and Clinical Factors. JAMA Netw Open. 2020;3(11):e2025074.
6. Mithal A, Bansal B, Kalra S. Gestational diabetes in India: Science and society. Indian J Endocrinol Metab. 2015;19(6):701-4.

2

CHAPTER

Pregnancy: A Diabetogenic State

INTRODUCTION

Pregnancy is a state of increased nutritional demands. Multiple physiologic and metabolic changes happen in pregnancy to meet the increased maternal demands and to adequately supply nutrients to the growing fetus. It starts as early as the first trimester of pregnancy and changes throughout pregnancy.

A normal pregnancy is characterized by increased insulin resistance, mild fasting hypoglycemia, and prolonged hyperglycemia after the meal.[1]

In early pregnancy, the basal blood glucose level and basal insulin levels remain unchanged and hence glucose tolerance is normal or slightly improved in the early trimester of pregnancy.[2] However, insulin sensitivity decreases with the advancing period of gestation to reach 50–60% of pregravid state by 34–36 weeks.[3] As a result of increased insulin resistance the basal as well as postprandial insulin secretion increases to almost twice the nonpregnant levels.[4] Pregnancy is characterized by hyperinsulinemia and euglycemia, a circumstance that fulfills Berson and Yalow's definition of insulin resistance, i.e., "a state in which greater than normal amounts of insulin are required to elicit a quantitatively normal response."[5] Studies with the euglycemic clamp technique suggest that the insulin resistance of pregnancy results from a target cell defect in insulin action beyond the initial step of binding to insulin receptors, a post-receptor defect of insulin action.[6]

Glucose being the preferred substrate for fetal source of energy leads to depletion of maternal reserves of glucose. The development of insulin resistance in early pregnancy limits the consumption of glucose by the mother and allows the transfer of glucose to the fetus.[7] Development of maternal insulin resistance during the third trimester of pregnancy results in a mild maternal carbohydrate intolerance in the last trimester.

Metabolic changes occurring in carbohydrate metabolism are largely influenced by high levels of maternal and placental hormones such as human chorionic somatomammotropin, estrogen, progesterone, prolactin, and cortisol.

PLACENTA

Early development of the placenta, is significantly influenced by the presence of insulin and tumor necrosis factor-α (TNF-α).

The various glucose transporters found at the maternal-fetal interface of the placenta are as follows:

- Glucose transporter 1 (GLUT1)—major glucose transporter in human placenta.
- GLUT3—high-affinity glucose transporter mainly found on fetoplacental endothelium.
- GLUT4—located in the stroma of placental villi.

The function of these transporters is regulated by various hormones and ambient glucose levels. The levels of glucose transporters are different in mothers with overt diabetes and gestational diabetes mellitus (GDM). As the pregnancy progresses, the placenta produces increasing amounts of diabetogenic hormones. Simultaneously, the adrenal glands are producing increased amounts of cortisol. All these hormones significantly impact the utilization of glucose thus sparing abundant glucose as substrate for the fetus.

During the third trimester of pregnancy, the mother's need for insulin increases progressively. In response to the increased demand for insulin, the normal β cells in the pancreatic islets of Langerhans undergo a 10–20% mass increase, which causes both hypertrophy and hyperplasia. On the other hand, for unknown reasons, it is manifested by increased insulin synthesis and secretion per cell.[7] However, gestational diabetes occurs when the pancreas is unable to meet these higher demands.[8]

Glyconeogenesis, the process by which glycogen is produced, is increased by 30% in the mother's liver due to insulin resistance. Insulin resistance limits the muscle's ability to consume glucose at the same time. Adipose tissue with insulin resistance has a sharp increase in lipolysis, which produces glycerol as a substrate for hepatic gluconeogenesis and fatty acids as an alternate fuel for mother consumption. Amino acids that are crucial for embryonic development are spared when the mother uses glycerol for gluconeogenesis.

To put it briefly, pregnancy changes the mother's metabolism such that the fetus receives the maximum amount of glucose transferred by the liver, the mother uses less glucose, and the amount of glucose converted to fat and glycogen is decreased. Despite her insulin resistance, the mother's fasting glucose levels decreased as a result of this reprogramming. However, the postprandial blood sugar level stays elevated for an extended amount of time.

Following a >12-hour fast, the mother's metabolism quickly shifts to using fat oxidation, increased ketone production, and the utilization of glycogenic or glycogenetic amino acids (amino acids like alanine and glutamic acid that can be converted to glucose). Acetone and β-hydroxybutyric acid are the main ketones or ketone bodies, which are metabolic byproducts of fatty acid catabolism for energy production. Hours before nonpregnant women fasted, lower plasma insulin and glucose levels as well as higher triglyceride-free levels of fatty acids and ketones are seen. Pregnant women can use fat reserves as a primary energy source, allowing the fetus to continue receiving glucose and amino acids due to the fasting metabolism that takes place during this time. Long-term usage of fetal ketone bodies is linked to a disruption of the newborn's physical and mental development. This is seen in women who do not control their diabetes well or in those who lose weight throughout pregnancy (either completely or for a portion of it).[9]

To recap, under the impact of numerous placental hormones, pregnancy is characterized by modest fasting hypoglycemia, postprandial hyperglycemia, and hyperinsulinemia.

REFERENCES

1. In: Iatrakis GM (Ed). Selected issues of obstetrics. Athens: Zevelekaki Publications; 2011. pp. 139-266.
2. Butte NF. Carbohydrate and lipid metabolism in pregnancy: Normal compared with gestational diabetes mellitus. Am J Clin Nutrition. 2000;71 (5 Suppl):1256S-61S.
3. Catalano PM, Tyzbir ED, Roman NM, Amini SB, Sims EA. Longitudinal changes in insulin release and insulin resistance in nonobese pregnant women. Am J Obstet Gynecol. 1991;165(6 Pt 1):1667-2.
4. Carpenter MW. Metabolic changes in gestational diabetes. Clin Perinatol. 1993;20(3):583-91.
5. Berson SA, Yalow RS. Insulin "antagonists" and insulin resistance. In: Ellenberg M, Rifkin H (Eds). Diabetes Mellitus: Theory and Practice. New York: McGraw-Hill; 1970. pp. 388-423.
6. Ryan EA, O'Sullivan MJ, Skyler JS. Insulin Action During Pregnancy. Studies with the Euglycemic Clamp Technique. Diabetes. 1985;34(4):380-9.
7. Liu LX, Arany Z. Maternal cardiac metabolism in pregnancy. Cardiovascular Research. 2014;101(4):545-53.
8. Vitoratos NA. Illustrated Obstetrics, 2nd edition. Bulgaria: Scientific Publications "Gr. Parisian"; 1996. pp. 33-6.
9. Lagowska K, Malinowska A, Zawieja B, Zawieja E. Improvement of glucose metabolism in pregnant women through probiotic supplementation depends on gestational diabetes status: meta-analysis. Scientific Reports. 2020;10: 17796.

3

CHAPTER

Pathophysiology of Gestational Diabetes Mellitus

INTRODUCTION

Gestational diabetes mellitus (GDM) is defined as glucose intolerance of various degrees that is first detected during pregnancy. It appears to result from the same broad spectrum of physiological and genetic abnormalities that characterize diabetes outside of pregnancy. Indeed, women with GDM are at high risk for having or developing diabetes when they are not pregnant. Gestational diabetes is type 2 diabetes mellitus unmasked or diagnosed first during the second trimester of pregnancy due to pregnancy-induced physiological changes in carbohydrate metabolism.

NORMAL PREGNANCY

Insulin resistance typically increases during pregnancy, starting around midpregnancy and reaching levels that are similar to those found in people with type 2 diabetes mellitus by the end of the third trimester. Insulin-desensitizing effects of placental hormones and increased maternal adiposities appear to be the cause of insulin resistance. Also, in response to the increased resistance, there is an increased secretion of insulin from the β-cells of the pancreas during pregnancy. The defining characteristic of normal glucose regulation during pregnancy is the robust plasticity of β-cell function in the face of progressive insulin resistance.

GESTATIONAL DIABETES

Gestational diabetes mellitus is a form of hyperglycemia unmasked during pregnancy. In general, the reason for hyperglycemia is an inadequate supply of insulin required to maintain normal blood sugar levels. Studies conducted before or after pregnancy, when women with prior GDM are usually more insulin resistant than normal women, often reveal insulin responses that are similar in the two groups or reduced only slightly in women with prior GDM.[1] However, women with a prior history of GDM show a significant defect in the function of β-cells of the pancreas. Possible causes of β-cell dysfunction could be: (1) Autoimmune, (2) monogenic, and (3) insulin resistance.

Autoimmune Diabetes and GDM

Type 1 diabetes results from autoimmune destruction of pancreatic β-cells. It accounts for roughly 5–10% of diabetes in the general population.[2]

Type 1 diabetes mellitus is characterized by antibodies directed against cells of pancreatic islets (anti-islet cell antibodies) or β-cell antigens [such as glutamic acid decarboxylase (GAD)]. Although, detailed physiological studies of these women are lacking, they most frequently have been found to have autoimmune destruction of pancreatic β-cells. The frequency of anti-islet cell and anti-GAD antibodies detected in GDM tends to parallel ethnical trends in the prevalence of type 1 diabetes.

Monogenic Diabetes and GDM

This type accounts for <10% of GDM cases.[3] Monogenic diabetes can present in two forms, one with mutations in autosomes and a second with mutations in mitochondrial deoxyribonucleic acid (DNA). Mutations in autosomes have an autosomal dominant inheritance pattern, commonly referred to as maturity-onset diabetes of the young (MODY). Patients with monogenic diabetes tend to be lean and do not show insulin resistance. Also, they are commonly seen at an early age. These women have abnormalities in the regulation of β-cell mass and/or function. Studies have shown that some women with MODY may have abnormalities in glucose-mediated insulin secretion. The various types of mutations seen in these women are found in genes coding for (1) glucokinase (MODY 2); (2) hepatocyte nuclear factor 1α (MODY 3); and (3) insulin promoter factor 1 (MODY 4).[4]

Insulin Resistance, ß-Cell Dysfunction, and GDM

Most women with GDM appear to have β-cell dysfunction on a background of chronic insulin resistance. As a result, pregnant women with GDM are more insulin-resistant than normal pregnant women. Differences in whole-body insulin sensitivity in the third trimester are small because of the significant effects of pregnancy on insulin resistance. However, accurate measurements of insulin sensitivity used in the third trimester have shown resistance to the ability of insulin to promote the utilization of glucose and inhibit glucose production and fatty acid levels in women with GDM.[5] After giving birth, when insulin resistance decreases, women with GDM are, on average, more insulin resistant than normal women. This finding, which has been consistent across studies in which whole-body insulin sensitivity has been measured directly, indicates that most women who develop GDM have chronic insulin resistance. Insulin sensitivity measurements performed in the same women before pregnancy, early in the second trimester, and in the third trimester have documented insulin resistance in both lean and obese women who go on to develop GDM.

Few of the biochemical mediators of chronic insulin resistance that accompany GDM and may contribute to the increased risk of type 2 diabetes have been studied. Women with GDM are more likely to be obese, so factors that promote obesity and/or the association of obesity with insulin resistance may be involved. Some studies have shown increased levels of leptin and inflammatory markers TNF-α and C-reactive protein and decreased levels of adiponectin in women with GDM.[6,7] Women with pre-existing gestational diabetes tend to have increased fat content in the liver and muscles. All of these findings are consistent with current understanding of some of the potential causes of obesity-related insulin resistance. Faulty mechanisms of the insulin signaling pathway, abnormal subcellular localization of GLUT4 transporters, reduced expression of peroxisome proliferator-activated receptor gamma (PPAR-γ), increased expression of the plasma cell membrane glycoprotein 1 (PC-1), and reduced insulin-mediated glucose transport have been found in skeletal muscle or fat cells of women with GDM.[8-10]

Glucose tolerance during early pregnancy is normal or slightly improved with normal peripheral (muscle) sensitivity to insulin and hepatic basal glucose production. These adaptive changes are due to the effect of pregnancy hormones namely, estrogen, progesterone, prolactin, and human chorionic somatomammotropin which cause pancreatic β-cell hyperplasia causing increased levels of insulin in early pregnancy. Insulin sensitivity of tissues changes throughout pregnancy with it being more in the first trimester and then decreasing sharply through the second and third trimesters. High levels of circulating insulin decrease the insulin-mediated glucose uptake in muscle and fat. This is a physiologic adaptation to preserve an adequate carbohydrate supply as a source of energy for the growing fetus. It appears that insulin secretion increases significantly in early pregnancy even before the development of insulin resistance. Studies have shown an increase in pancreatic β-cell area in pregnancy.

REFERENCES

1. Homko C, Sivan E, Chen X, Reece EA, Boden G. Insulin secretion during and after pregnancy in patients with gestational diabetes mellitus. J Clin Endocrinol Metab. 2001;86(2):568-73.
2. American Diabetes Association. Diagnosis and classification of diabetes mellitus. Diabetes Care. 2004;27(Suppl 1):S5-10.
3. Weng J, Ekelund M, Lehto M, Li H, Ekberg G, Frid A, et al. Screening for MODY mutations, GAD antibodies, and type 1 diabetes—associated HLA genotypes in women with gestational diabetes mellitus. Diabetes Care. 2002;25(1):68-71.
4. Kousta E, Ellard S, Allen LI, Saker PJ, Huxtable SJ, Hattersley AT, et al. Glucokinase mutations in a phenotypically selected multiethnic group of women with a history of gestational diabetes. Diabet Med. 2001;18(8):683-4.
5. Xiang AH, Peters RK, Trigo E, Kjos SL, Lee WP, Buchanan TA. Multiple metabolic defects during late pregnancy in women at high risk for type 2 diabetes mellitus. Diabetes. 1999;48(4):848-54.
6. Retnakaran R, Hanley AJ, Raif N, Connelly PW, Sermer M, Zinman B. C-reactive protein and gestational diabetes: the central role of maternal obesity. J Clin Endocrinol. Metab. 2003;88(8):3507-12.

7. Retnakaran R, Hanley AJ, Raif N, Connelly PW, Sermer M, Zinman B. Reduced adiponectin concentration in women with gestational diabetes: a potential factor in progression to type 2 diabetes. Diabetes Care. 2004;27(3):799-800.
8. Damm P, Handberg A, Kühl C, Beck-Nielsen H, Mølsted-Pedersen L. Insulin receptor binding and tyrosine kinase activity in skeletal muscle from normal pregnant women and women with gestational diabetes. Obstet Gynecol. 1993;82(2):251-9.
9. Catalano PM, Nizielski SE, Shao J, Preston L, Qiao L, Friedman JE. Downregulated IRS-1 and PPARgamma in obese women with gestational diabetes: relationship to FFA during pregnancy. Am J Physiol. 2002;282(3):E522-33.
10. Garvey WT, Maianu L, Zhu JH, Hancock JA, Golichowski AM. Multiple defects in the adipocyte glucose transport system cause cellular insulin resistance in gestational diabetes. Heterogeneity in the number and a novel abnormality in subcellular localization of GLUT4 glucose transporters. Diabetes. 1993;42(12):1773-85.

CHAPTER 4

Obesity and Chronic Diabetes

INTRODUCTION

Diabetes is known to be a noncommunicable disease. Owing to the excessive consumption of high-fat foods, lack of physical activity and an increasing trend of sedentary work profile the incidence and prevalence of obesity has nearly doubled worldwide. According to reports of studies conducted in the age group of 18 years and above, >39% of adults were overweight while 13% were obese. According to the World Health Organization (WHO), 41 million children under the age of 5 years were either overweight or obese.[1] Obesity not only causes physical disabilities but also has a significant impact on the psychological health of the individual. According to WHO 44% of patients with diabetes, 23% of patients with ischemic heart disease, and 7–41% of patients with cancers have obesity as the comorbidity.[2] If timely interventions are not carried out then the prevalence of diabetes in obese individuals is expected to double to 300 million by 2025.[3]

Type 1 diabetes is more commonly seen in children and adults during their forties. The main pathophysiology for type 1 diabetes is pancreatic cell destruction. The etiology in the majority of cases is infectious or environmental. Autoimmunity is an important mechanism of pathophysiology for diabetes. In genetically susceptible individuals there is an exaggerated immune response against beta cells of the pancreas.[4] Antibodies against islet cells and insulin are commonly found in patients with type 1 diabetes. While type 1 diabetes has low levels of insulin and hence glucose utilization, type 2 diabetes is characterized by peripheral insulin resistance. Type 2 diabetes develops in those overweight and obese patients in whom the pancreas fails to secrete sufficient amounts of insulin to overcome insulin resistance. Insulin resistance causes decreased glucose uptake and increased breakdown of fats leading to elevated levels of fatty acids in the plasma. Diabetes thus affects carbohydrate, protein, and fat metabolism.

OBESITY AND INSULIN RESISTANCE

By releasing nonesterified fatty acids and secreting hormones, glycerol, and other chemicals such as leptin, cytokines, adiponectin, and proinflammatory compounds, adipose tissue influences metabolism in the body. These compounds are secreted at higher rates in obese people. Research indicates that while peripheral insulin uptake improves with the administration of antilipolytic medications, insulin resistance rises following the release of high concentrations of non-esterified fatty acids. Body fat distribution is another important component that determines insulin sensitivity. Body mass index (BMI) and variations in body fat distribution are linked to insulin resistance. Insulin sensitivity is higher in those with a more peripheral distribution of fat than in people with a more central distribution of fat (i.e., in the belly and chest area).[5]

The differences in the metabolic effects of subcutaneous and intra-abdominal fat can be partially explained by variations in the location of adipose tissue. The genes that secrete certain types of proteins and those that are in charge of producing energy are more closely linked to intra-abdominal fat. More adiponectin is secreted by omental adipocytes than by adipocytes coming from the subcutaneous layer. Furthermore, there is a negative correlation between elevated body weight and the amount released by these omental adipocytes.

Additionally, abdominal fat is thought to be more lipolytic than subcutaneous fat, and it also reacts more slowly to insulin's antilipolytic effects. For these reasons, intra-abdominal fat plays a larger role in the development of insulin resistance and ultimately diabetes.

PREPREGNANCY BODY MASS INDEX AND DIABETES

The development of gestational diabetes mellitus is significantly increased in women who are obese before becoming pregnant, with an increased risk of four and eight times, respectively, as compared to women of normal weight. Women should not only maintain a healthy weight before becoming pregnant but also gain the recommended amount of weight during the pregnancy based on their BMI category.

Women are classified into four groups based on their prepregnancy BMI: underweight (BMI: <18.5 kg/m^2), normal weight (BMI: 18.5–24.9 kg/m^2), overweight (BMI: 25.0–29.9 kg/m^2), or obese (BMI: ≥ 30.0 kg/m^2). As per the American College of Obstetricians and Gynecologists (ACOG) (ACOG Committee opinion no. 548, 2013), excessive weight gain is defined as the total gestational weight gain above the maximum limit for each BMI class, which is 18.0, 16.0, 11.5, and 9.0 kg for prepregnancy underweight, normal weight, overweight, and obese mothers, respectively.

Obese women who put on too much weight while pregnant have a higher chance of having obese children. According to studies, maternal glucose homeostasis status or weight increase during pregnancy were not as powerful perinatal predictors of high BMI in childhood as prepregnancy obesity was. In a similar vein, postpartum weight retention is more common in women who gain more weight during pregnancy than is advised.

Fetal hyperinsulinemia can be caused by maternal insulin resistance and the ensuing hyperglycemia, which can result in excessive fetal development linked to macrosomia and increased obesity. Even in cases where glucose levels are properly managed, recent research indicates that maternal hypertriglyceridemia brought on by insulin resistance may potentially play a role in larger babies and higher levels of obesity. The long-term obesity of the offspring may be impacted by excessive adiposity at birth. Additionally, there is proof that elevated levels of leptin in the mother affect how her offspring regulate their appetite and maintain metabolic homeostasis. A major modulator of metabolic balance is leptin, a hormone released by adipose tissue at levels that are directly associated with body fat stores. Pregnancy-related hyperleptinemia may lessen the sensitivity of growing fetal organs, especially the hypothalamus, to leptin. Leptin functions to limit food intake and increase energy expenditure by acting on the hypothalamus; hence, irreversible modifications in leptin sensitivity could have long-term ramifications for energy balance in offspring, extending the cycle of obesity.

REFERENCES

1. World Health Organization. (2024). Obesity and Overweight. [online] Available from www.who.int/mediacentre/factsheets/fs311/en/ [Last accessed November, 2024].
2. Frühbeck G, Toplak H, Woodward E, Yumuk V, Maislos M, Oppert JM; Executive Committee of the European Association for the Study of Obesity. Obesity: the gateway to ill health — an EASO position statement on a rising public health, clinical and scientific challenge in Europe. Obes Facts. 2013;6(2):117-20.
3. Dyson PA. The therapeutics of lifestyle management on obesity. Diabetes Obes Metab. 2010;12(11):941-6.
4. Hutton JC, Davidson HW. Cytokine-induced dicing and splicing in the beta-cell and the immune response in type 1 diabetes. Diabetes. 2010;59(2):335-6.
5. Karpe F, Dickmann JR, Frayn KN. Fatty acids, obesity, and insulin resistance: time for a reevaluation. Diabetes. 2011;60(10):2441-9.

5

CHAPTER

How Gestational Diabetes Mellitus Affects Mother and Fetus?

INTRODUCTION

Gestational diabetes mellitus is a form of type 2 diabetes mellitus (DM) characterized by increased insulin resistance and hyperglycemia in the presence of normal or high insulin levels. The phenomenon of insulin resistance is because of the diabetogenic effect of pregnancy-related hormones which either aggravate the preexisting diabetic condition or unmasks the latent diabetic state. There is a serious concern about the future development of type 2 DM in the mother as well as the baby. A systematic review conducted by Kim et al. concluded that the progression to type 2 DM increased steeply within the first 5 years after delivery and then appeared to plateau and that fasting hyperglycemia was the most important risk factor for the development of future diabetes.[1]

MATERNAL EFFECTS

Long-standing diabetes results in microvascular and macrovascular complications eventually leading to end organ damage.

DIABETIC NEPHROPATHY

Long-standing uncontrolled diabetes is the most common cause of end-stage renal disease. Approximately 5% of pregnant women with diabetes have renal involvement—White class F.[2] It increases the risk of development of preeclampsia, fetal growth restriction, and consequential iatrogenic preterm birth. **Table 1** summarizes the natural history of the progression of diabetic nephropathy. Diabetic nephropathy begins with the appearance of clinically detectable proteins in the urine in the form of microalbuminuria 30–300 mg/24 h of albumin which develops 5 years after the onset of diabetes. Over the next 5–10 years overt proteinuria—urine albumin >300 mg/24 h develops in patients with uncontrolled blood sugar levels. This progression can be prevented by optimal glycemic control. Hypertension starts manifesting at this stage. All pregestational diabetics as well as newly diagnosed gestational diabetic mothers should therefore be screened with urine protein test at their first antenatal visit. Proteinuria, being a common symptom of preeclampsia as well as diabetic nephropathy, is essential to monitor blood pressure regularly in patients with overt diabetes.

TABLE 1: The stages of development of diabetic nephropathy.

*Estimated glomerular filtration rate (GFR)**		*Albuminuria*	*Serum creatinine (µmol/L) (mg/dL)*	*Blood pressure (mm Hg)*	*Renal structural changes*
I stage	≥90	Normoalbuminuria	Normal [<100 (<1.1)]	Normal <130/80	Glomerular hypertrophy
II stage	60–89	Intermittent micro-albuminuria	Normal	Normal <130/80	Increased glomerular basement membrane thickness
III stage	30–59	Persistent microalbuminuria	100–124 (1.1–1.4)	Slightly elevated (130–139)	Decrease in and changes in glomerular epithelial cells
IV stage	15–29	Macroalbuminuria (≥300 mg/24 h)	Moderately increased (azotemia)	Moderately increased (140–159)	Glomerulosclerosis and tubulointerstitial fibrosis
V stage	<15 or dialysis	Macroalbuminuria (can decrease, pseudonormalization)	Markedly increased (uremia)	Markedly increased (≥160/110)	

*Glomerular filtration ratio estimated as mL/min/m^2

Studies have shown that pregnancy was not associated with the development and progression of diabetic nephropathy in women with normal renal function or mild renal dysfunction however women with moderate to severe nephropathy may progress to end-stage renal disease (ESRD).[3] Renal dysfunction is correlated with poor perinatal outcomes.

Angiotensin-converting enzyme (ACE) inhibitors or angiotensin II receptor blockers are recommended for treatment before conception and postdelivery; however, they are contraindicated in pregnancy as they are associated with fetal proximal renal tubular agenesis and oligohydramnios. Alternatively, pregnancy-safe drugs such as labetalol and alpha methyldopa should be started as soon as pregnancy is detected. Optimal glycemic control and treatment of coexisting hypertension can delay the progression to ESRD.

DIABETIC RETINOPATHY

Diabetic retinopathy is the most frequent cause of new cases of blindness among adults aged 20–74 years in developed countries. Poor glycemic control, longer duration of diabetes, greater fall in blood glucose in early pregnancy, dyslipidemia, and raised blood pressure have been identified as risk factors for the progression of retinopathy during pregnancy.[4] A wide variety of lesions have been reported under the spectrum of diabetic retinopathy. The staging of diabetic retinopathy is depicted in **Figure 1**.

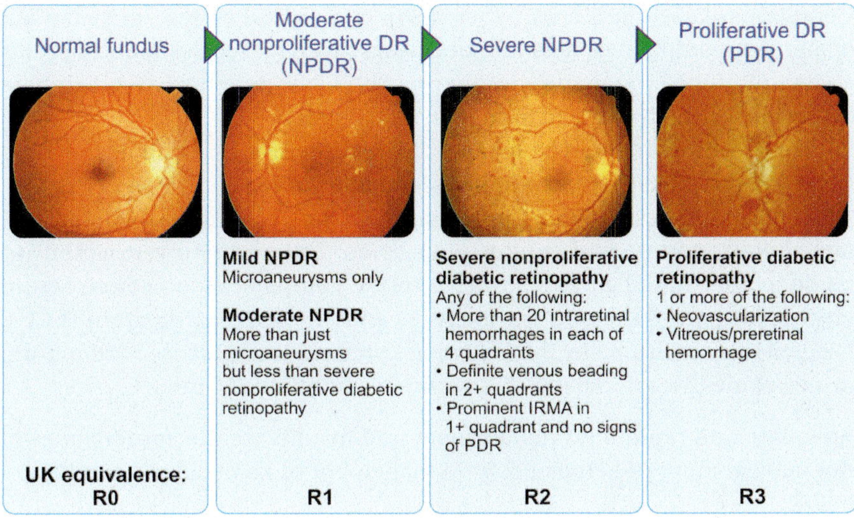

Fig. 1: Staging of diabetic retinopathy according to the American Academy of Ophthalmology.

In known diabetic females, a fundoscopic eye check-up is recommended before conception, at the first antenatal visit, and at 28 weeks if all previous examinations are normal. In case of preexisting lesion, a repeat examination should be done at 16–20 weeks.[5] Retinopathy worsens during pregnancy hence a pre-existing proliferative retinopathy should be detected at prepregnancy check-ups and ideally treated by laser photocoagulation before conception. The nonproliferative stage of retinopathy can be managed by tight glycemic control however, proliferative retinopathy is treated by pan photo coagulation which can be safely carried out during pregnancy. Diabetic macular edema needs to be controlled by focal or grid laser coagulation. Diabetic retinopathy is not a contraindication for vaginal delivery. But in cases of proliferative retinopathy, labor may cause an increase in intraocular pressure resulting in sudden intravitreal hemorrhage due to rupture of vessels. Hence, in such patients with untreated proliferative retinopathy, caesarean section is a safe mode of delivery. However, the decision regarding the mode of delivery needs to be individualized. Women with PDR in pregnancy should have ophthalmological follow-up for at least 6 months following the birth of the baby.[6]

DIABETIC KETOACIDOSIS

Diabetic ketoacidosis is a life-threatening complication of DM occurring mostly in type 1 DM, but rarely in type 2 diabetics. It is characterized by hyperglycemia, dehydration, and acidosis with ketonemia and ketonuria. Maternal mortality due to this complication is reported to be 5–15%.

Conditions like febrile illness, hyperemesis or diarrheal disease, dehydration, insulin noncompliance, beta mimetic drugs given for tocolysis, and steroids given to induce lung maturation in preterm labor patients can precipitate ketoacidosis which can lead to sudden fetal death.

These mothers should be managed in an intensive care unit in consultation with a physician with continuous fetal monitoring.

The patient presents with signs of dehydration, tachycardia, hypotension, tachypnoea, and mental confusion or coma. Laboratory investigations to be done are—blood glucose, urine ketones, complete blood count, serum electrolytes, arterial blood gas analysis, and an electrocardiogram (ECG). Diagnosis is confirmed by the following criteria: Blood glucose >250 mg/dL, urine ketones 3+, arterial pH <7.3, serum bicarbonate <15 mEq/L.

Adequate and rapid fluid replacement and insulin are the cornerstones of the management of ketoacidosis. Management of ketoacidosis is outlined below:

- A comatose patient may need ventilator support.
- Monitoring of pulse, blood pressure, capillary blood glucose, input and output, urine ketones, blood gas analysis, and serum electrolytes.
- A wide-bore intravenous access must be secured.
- Estimated fluid deficit in these patients is around 100 mL/kg, i.e., 5–6 L. Fluid correction must be rapid in the first 4 hours, i.e., 500–1,000 mL/h followed by 250 mL/h till pulse and blood pressure are normalized. Initial replacement is using normal saline which is late switched over to 5% dextrose once blood glucose falls below 250 mg/dL.
- Insulin therapy is started using 0.2 U/kg intravenous bolus followed by 0.1 U/kg/h in normal saline. If the blood glucose does not fall by 30 in the first 3 hours, then the drip rate is doubled.
- Hypokalemia $K^+ < 4$ mEq/L is corrected with 30 mEq/h KCl.
- Bicarbonate is required if pH is <7.1. Add one ampoule, i.e., 44 mEq to 1 L of 0.45% normal saline.
- Treatment of the cause is important.
- Fetal well-being is assessed by cardiotocography. Nonreassuring patterns will generally improve once the maternal condition is stabilized.

DIABETIC NEUROPATHY

Cardiac autonomic neuropathy is a common dysfunction in patients with long-term DM and is associated with inadequate glycemic control and the duration of diabetes.[7] GDM is considered to be pretype 2 DM. These patients show subclinical inflammatory processes and associated endothelial dysfunction. Hyperglycemia due to abnormal glucose metabolism is also associated with chronic idiopathic axonal polyneuropathy (burning feet syndrome). Various studies have shown an association between the development of diabetic foot syndrome and diabetic peripheral neuropathy with female sex.[8] Therefore women with GDM should be warned about the signs of peripheral neuropathy namely, numbness of feet, burning or pricking sensation over feet, dryness or callus formation, pain while walking, and ingrown toenails.

Fetal Effects

Congenital Malformations

The incidence of major malformations in GDM mothers is similar to non-diabetics because the blood sugar level is normal during the period of organogenesis. However, women with Pregestational diabetes have a two to ninefold higher risk of having babies with birth defects, with a prevalence of birth defects of 2.7–18.6%, compared with the healthy population having a prevalence of birth defects of 2–3%.[9] Poor glycemic control during the critical period of organogenesis is the major determinant of congenital malformation. Studies have shown that maternal diabetes triggers stress responses leading to aberrant signal transduction pathways, this in turn increases the production of cellular reactive oxygen species and simultaneously impairs endogenous cellular antioxidant capacity, leading to an overall oxidative stress in the embryo.[10] There is accelerated apoptosis of growing cells in the embryo leading to structural defects.

Levels of glycated hemoglobin (HbA1C) correlate well with the risk of congenital malformation.

- HbA1C <7%—risk of anomalies no greater than nondiabetic mother
- 7–8.5%—5% risk
- >10%—risk rises to 22%

However recent study findings might implicate that for prevention of congenital malformations and macrosomia in diabetic pregnancies, HbA1c should be below 5.0% in the first trimester of pregnancy and below 6.0% in the third trimester.[11] The most commonly affected systems are the central nervous system and the cardiovascular system.

- *Central nervous system (CNS):* Anencephaly, holoprosencephaly, occipital encephalocele, and meningomyelocele.
- *Cardiovascular system (CVS):* Transposition of great vessels, ventricular and atrial septal defects, tetralogy of Fallot, hypoplastic left heart
- *Skeletal system:* Caudal regression syndrome and spinal defects
- *Renal system:* Renal agenesis, polycystic kidneys, and ureteric duplication
- *Gastrointestinal (GI) system:* Duodenal atresia, anorectal malformations, and omphalocele
- *Musculoskeletal system:* Arthrogryposis and hypoplastic femur
- *Functional:* Intraventricular septal hypertrophy, small left colon syndrome

All mothers with preexisting DM must be counseled regarding the risks of anomalies based on their glycemic control. Mothers with poor glycemic control and high HbA1C values should be warned about the possible anomalies and the decision to continue pregnancy should be at her discretion. Early screening for congenital anomalies by an expert sinologist should be offered to all diabetic mothers.

SPONTANEOUS ABORTION

Poor glycemic control in the first trimester in pre-gestational diabetic mothers increases the likelihood of spontaneous abortion.[12] The most probable cause is major malformations incompatible with life. A good pre and periconceptional glycemic control can reduce the risk of abortions.

PRETERM DELIVERY

Poor control of blood sugar levels during pregnancy is associated with both spontaneous and indicated preterm delivery. Hyperglycemia directly induces endothelial dysfunction and increased oxidative stress leading to blunted nitric oxide-dependent vasodilatation. During pregnancy, decreased synthesis of nitric oxide in the uterus is associated with the initiation of labor in animals, and nitric oxide is a uterine relaxant. These observations suggest that strict glycemic control might reduce the rate of preterm delivery.

A study by Lepercq et al. showed that the rate of preterm delivery remains high in women with type 1 DM.[13] Because poor glycemic control was a risk factor for both outcomes, part of preterm delivery might be preventable.

ALTERED FETAL GROWTH

Birth weight >90th percentile or >2 SD for the gestational age or macrosomia >4,000 g is the hallmark of poorly controlled maternal diabetes. The amount of fat deposited in the fetus is correlated with the fasting glucose levels in the mother. Early treatment to control blood sugar levels prevents pancreatic beta cell hyperplasia in the fetus.

The disproportion between the head and the shoulder girdle increases the risk of shoulder dystocia, obstructed labor, birth injuries to the baby, perineal injuries to the mother, and increased incidence of instrumental delivery and caesarean section.

SUDDEN UNEXPLAINED FETAL DEMISE

The key pathway leading to intrauterine fetal death is chronic hypoxia. Fetal hyperglycemia results in fetal pancreatic beta cell hyperplasia and hence hyperinsulinemia. Increased levels of insulin lead to increased oxygen consumption and decreased arterial oxygen. Fetal hyperglycemia has also been associated with cardiomyopathy secondary to myocardial ischemia.

POLYHYDRAMNIOS

Polyhydramnios is defined as a four-quadrant amniotic fluid index (AFI) >24 cm or a single maximum vertical pocket >8 cm. As per the literature, approximately 60% of polyhydramnios are idiopathic; 20% of cases can be attributed to poorly controlled or undiagnosed diabetes, and the remainder of cases are associated with fetal anomalies.[14] Several adverse outcomes have been associated with polyhydramnios including preterm labor, rupture of membranes, and cord prolapse. Queenan first reported the association between diabetes during pregnancy and polyhydramnios in 1971. He found that approximately one in four cases of polyhydramnios were due to diabetes.[14] There has not been any significant increase in adverse perinatal outcomes with an isolated finding of polyhydramnios other than iatrogenic preterm delivery due to the nonavailability of an effective modality of fetal surveillance in these mothers.

NEONATAL EFFECTS

- *Respiratory distress syndrome (RDS):* Poor glycemic control delays lung maturity which manifests as RDS in newborns. This risk is low after 38 completed weeks of pregnancy. Hence every attempt should be made to prolong pregnancy till 38 weeks. In case of premature termination of pregnancy, corticosteroids should be given to the mother with close supervision of blood sugar levels.
- *Hypoglycemia:* It occurs as a consequence of fetal hyperinsulinemia in the newborn immediately following delivery. Neonatal hypoglycemia is defined as blood sugar <40 mg/dL at term during the first 12 hours of life. A neonate with hypoglycemia presents with lethargy, poor feeding, and seizures. Preterm neonates are at higher risk of hypoglycemia as compared to term neonates.
- *Hypocalcemia*: Neonatal hypocalcemia is total serum calcium <8 mg/dL in term infants and <7 mg/dL in preterm infants. This is a consequence of maternal hypomagnesemia caused by excessive renal losses in poorly controlled diabetic mothers.
- *Hyperbilirubinemia*: Usually seen from the second day onward. It is linked to an immature hepatic bilirubin conjugation system and neonatal polycythemia. Birth trauma leading to hematoma formation further worsens the condition.
- *Polycythemia*: It is defined as venous hematocrit of >65%. Fetal tissue hypoxia stimulates fetal erythropoietin secretion leading to polycythemia. The consequences of this response are increased viscosity of blood, poor circulation, ischemia, and microthrombi formation leading to infarction in vital organs.

- *Impaired cognitive development*: The rapid fetal brain development coincides with the development of GDM in the mother thus affecting the baby's neurocognitive development.
- *Development of diabetes in the future*: Neonates exposed to hyperglycemia in utero is at increased risk of obesity and type 2 DM in childhood or adulthood.

REFERENCES

1. Kim C, Newton KM, Knopp RH. Gestational diabetes and the incidence of type 2 diabetes: a systematic review. Diabetes Care. 2002;25(10):1862-8.
2. Hanson UI, Persson B. Outcome of pregnancies complicated by type 1 insulin-dependent diabetes in Sweden: acute pregnancy complications, neonatal mortality and morbidity. Am J Perinatol. 1993;10(04):330-3.
3. Young EC, Pires MLE, Marques LPJ, de Oliveira JEP, Zajdenverg L. Effects of pregnancy on the onset and progression of diabetic nephropathy and of diabetic nephropathy on pregnancy outcomes. Diabetes Metab Syndr. 2011;5(3):137-42.
4. Axer-Siegel R, Hod M, Fink-Cohen S, Kramer M, Weinberger D, Schindel B, et al. Diabetic retinopathy during pregnancy. Ophthalmology. 1996;103(11):1815-9.
5. National Collaborating Centre for Women's and Children's Health (UK). Diabetes in Pregnancy: Management of Diabetes and Its Complications from Preconception to the Postnatal Period. London: RCOG Press; 2008.
6. Ghanchi F; Diabetic Retinopathy Guidelines Working Group. The Royal College of Ophthalmologists' clinical guidelines for diabetic retinopathy: a summary. Eye (Lond). 2013;27(2):285-7.
7. Singh JP, Larson MG, O'Donnell CJ, Wilson PF, Tsuji H, Lloyd-Jones DM, et al. Association of hyperglycemia with reduced heart rate variability (The Framingham Heart Study). Am J Cardiol. 2000;86(3):309-12.
8. Solanki JD, Makwana AH, Mehta HB, Gokhle PA, Shah CJ, Hathilla PB. Assessment of Ankle Brachial Index in Diabetic patients in Urban area of West India. Int J Basic Appl Physiol. 2012;1:114-9.
9. Temple R, Aldridge V, Greenwood R, Heyburn P, Sampson M, Stanley K. Association between outcome of pregnancy and glycaemic control in early pregnancy in type 1 diabetes: population based study. BMJ. 2002;325(7375):1275-6.
10. Reece EA, Ma XD, Zhao Z, Wu YK, Dhanasekaran D. Aberrant patterns of cellular communication in diabetes-induced embryopathy in rats: II, apoptotic pathways. Am J Obstet Gynecol. 2005;192(3):967-72.
11. Radder JK, van Roosmalen J. HbA1c in healthy, pregnant women. Neth J Med. 2005;63(7):256-9.
12. Wright AD, Nicholson HO, Pollock A, Taylor KG, Betts S. Spontaneous abortion and diabetes mellitus. Postgrad Med J. 1983;59(691):295-8.
13. Lepercq J, Coste J, Theau A, Dubois-Laforgue D, Timsit J. Factors associated with preterm delivery in women with type 1 diabetes: a cohort study. Diabetes Care. 2004;27(12):2824-8.
14. Moore LE. Amount of polyhydramnios attributable to diabetes may be less than previously reported. World J Diabetes. 2017;8(1):7-10.

6 CHAPTER

The Dilemmas in Screening Methods

INTRODUCTION

Over the last few years, there have been different opinions regarding the universal acceptability of screening and diagnostic techniques used for gestational diabetes mellitus (GDM) due to differences in population risks, cost-effectiveness, and lack of evidence.

EVOLUTION OF SCREENING METHODS OVER THE LAST 50 YEARS

1964, O'Sullivan and Mahan

The duo devised this method for diagnosing GDM in pregnancy based on the woman's risk of developing type 2 diabetes mellitus in her future life. The diagnostic criteria were given by performing a 100 g oral glucose tolerance test on 752 females with measurement of whole blood glucose at 1, 2, and 3 hours.[1] Woman was diagnosed with GDM if two or more blood glucose values were met or exceeded. The test was costly and was too tedious to perform as it required multiple blood sample collection.

1973, O'Sullivan

The first glucose challenge test (GCT) using 50 g glucose followed by whole blood glucose examination after 1 hour was suggested. Using 130 mg/dL as the upper limit, the sensitivity of the test is 79% and specificity is 87%.[2] Women whose blood glucose levels exceeded the screening threshold were further subjected to undergo a 100 g, 3 hours oral glucose tolerance test (OGTT). In this subsequent approach, women who have two or more abnormal values at fasting, 1 hour, 2 hours, and 3 hours postglucose consumption were diagnosed to have GDM. The disadvantage of this test was that the positive and negative predictive values were dependent on the prevalence of GDM in the population.

1979, National Diabetes Data Group

The US National Diabetes Data Group (NDDG) used the 3-hour 100 g OGTT but instead of using whole blood glucose levels, they used venous plasma glucose levels as they gave values 11% higher than those of whole blood.[3] the disadvantages of this test were the same as those of the test given by O'Sullivan and Mahan.

1982, Carpenter and Coustan

Glucose estimation was now being done using specific enzyme assays instead of the calorimetric method used earlier. This method enabled Carpenter and Coustan to lower the cut-off values set by NDDG for the diagnosis of GDM.

1999, World Health Organization

According to the recommendations given by the World Health Organization (WHO) in the year 1999, a single cut-off value was considered for the diagnosis of GDM and diabetes. After overnight fasting the woman was subjected to an oral glucose load of 75 g and plasma glucose value was checked after 2 hours of the glucose load. A woman with a value >140 mg/dL was diagnosed to be having GDM and those with a value >200 mg/dL were diagnosed with overt diabetes during pregnancy.[4] Even this test did not consider adverse perinatal outcomes but only the future risk of developing diabetes in the mother.

2006, Diabetes in Pregnancy Study Group India

World Health Organization's recommendation for the 75 g glucose test required long fasting hours before the glucose challenge which caused many women to opt out of the test. Therefore, in the year 2006, the Diabetes in Pregnancy Study Group India (DIPSI) came up with a modification in the recommendation which involved a 75 g glucose challenge and measurement of venous plasma glucose in a nonfasting state at 24–28 weeks of pregnancy irrespective of the last meal consumption.[5]

The Hyperglycemia and Adverse Pregnancy Outcomes (HAPO) Study conducted in the year 2008 showed that hyperglycemia during early pregnancy was associated with adverse neonatal outcomes.[6] With an intention to mitigate the adverse effects observed in the HAPO study, the International Association of Diabetes and Pregnancy Study Groups (IADPSG) recommended a one-step 75 g OGTT test and lowered the diagnostic cut-off of the OGTT (92, 180, and 153 mg/dL at fasting, 1 hour and 2 hours postprandial) in 2010.[7] In this approach, GDM is diagnosed in women who have one abnormal value. **Table 1** summarizes various diagnostic criteria used for the diagnosis of GDM.

WHO SHOULD BE SCREENED?

The American College of Obstetricians and Gynecologists (ACOG) recommends considering early screening in pregnancy if:

The patient is overweight with a BMI of 25 (23 in Asian Americans), and one of the following:

- Physical inactivity
- Known impaired glucose metabolism

TABLE 1: Diagnostic criteria for diagnosis of GDM.

	O'Sullivan (1964) (100 g OGTT)	*NDDG (75 g OGTT)*	*Carpenter and Coustan (100 g OGTT)*	*IADPSG (75 g OGTT)*
Number of abnormal values required for diagnosis	>2	>2	>2	>1
Fasting (mg/dL)	90	105	95	92
After 1 hour (mg/dL)	165	190	180	180
After 2 hours (mg/dL)	145	165	155	153
After 3 hours (mg/dL)	125	145	140	

(GDM: gestational diabetes mellitus; IADPSG: International Association of the Diabetes and Pregnancy Study Groups; NDDG: National Diabetes Data Group; OGTT: oral glucose tolerance test)

- Previous pregnancy history of:
  - GDM
  - Macrosomia (≥4,000 g)
  - Stillbirth
- Hypertension (140/90 mm Hg or being treated for hypertension)
- High-density-lipoprotein cholesterol ≤35 mg/dL (0.90 mmol/L)
- Fasting triglyceride ≥250 mg/dL (2.82 mmol/L)
- Polycystic ovary syndrome, acanthosis nigricans, nonalcoholic steatohepatitis, morbid obesity, and other conditions associated with insulin resistance
- Glycated hemoglobin HgbA1C ≥5.7%, impaired glucose tolerance or impaired fasting glucose. If HgbA1C >6.5%, diagnosis of pregestational diabetes is met and GCT/GTT not needed
- Cardiovascular disease
- Family history of diabetes—first-degree relative (parent or sibling)
- Ethnicity of African American, American Indian, Asian American, Hispanic, Latina, or Pacific Islander.

INDIAN GUIDELINES

Consequently, in 2014, keeping in view the contrasts in national and worldwide guidelines for diagnosing GDM, the Government of India (GOI) defined its criteria based on the DIPSI guidelines **(Flowchart 1)**. They suggested widespread screening of all Indian pregnant females twice amid their whole antenatal period by taking after one-step strategy utilizing 2-hour 75 g OGTT independent of their last meal timings. The reason for universal screening was to give the benefit of early diagnosis to all women who walk into the antenatal clinic unaware of their pre-pregnancy blood glucose levels. This circumstance essentially holds genuine in India which positions

Flowchart 1: Diagnosis and management of GDM technical and operational guidelines (Maternal Health Division, Ministry of Health and Family Welfare of India).

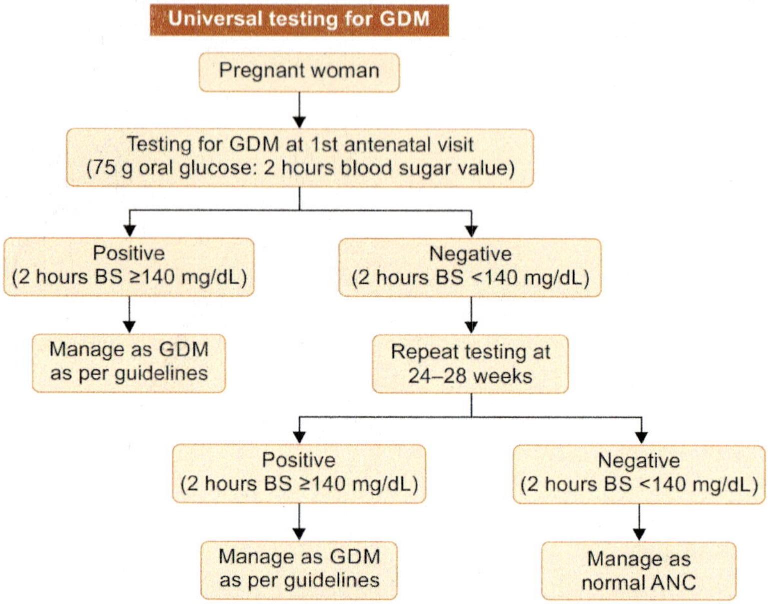

(ANC: antenatal care; GDM: gestational diabetes mellitus)

most noteworthy among South-Asian nations about the predominance of GDM. The guideline suggests consumption of 75 g anhydrous glucose dissolved in 300 mL water independent of the last meal timings. The intake is to be completed within 5 minutes. In case vomiting happens within 30 minutes of glucose intake, the test should be retaken on another day. But if it happens after 30 minutes, the test proceeds. The primary test is to be done early in pregnancy and then between 24 and 28 weeks of pregnancy with a minimum gap of 4 weeks between the two tests. On the off chance that the woman presents past 28 weeks of gestation, then only one test is to be done at the primary contact. The national rules moreover order the accessibility of plasma-calibrated glucometers at all antenatal clinics located at medical colleges, district hospitals and other Comprehensive Emergency Obstetric Care Services (CEmOC) centers to assess blood glucose 2 hours after the oral glucose consumption rather than semiautoanalyzer or autoanalyzer. This can be to guarantee immediate interpretation of results which can be made accessible to the subject on the same day.[8]

Since the introduction of screening and diagnostic methods for GDM, there have been multiple studies and criteria given by the studies. However, not all criteria have been economical and accurate. Considering the adverse effects of diabetes in pregnancy, it is of utmost importance to diagnose the disease at the earliest. However, the exact lower value to be used is still of debate whether it is to be clinical or to be governed by health economics. To conclude, the diagnostic criteria should be cost-effective as well as most accurate for the population it is being used for.

REFERENCES

1. O'sullivan JB, Mahan CM. Criteria for the oral glucose tolerance test in pregnancy. Diabetes. 1964;13:278-85.
2. O'Sullivan JB, Mahan CM, Charles D, Dandrow RV. Screening criteria for high-risk gestational diabetic patients. Am J Obstet Gynecol. 1973;116(7):895-900.
3. National Diabetes Data Group. Classification and diagnosis of diabetes mellitus and other categories of glucose intolerance. National Diabetes Data Group. Diabetes. 1979;28(12):1039-57.
4. World Health Organization. Definition, Diagnosis and Classification of Diabetes Mellitus and Its Complications. Part 1: diagnosis and classification of diabetes mellitus provisional report of a WHO consultation. Diabet Med. 1998;15(7):539-53.
5. Seshiah V, Das AK, Balaji V, Joshi SR, Parikh MN, Gupta S. Gestational diabetes mellitus—guidelines. J Assoc Physicians India. 2006;54:622-8.
6. HAPO Study Cooperative Research Group; Metzger BE, Lowe LP, Dyer AR, Trimble ER, Chaovarindr U, et al. Hyperglycemia and adverse pregnancy outcomes. N Engl J Med. 2008;358(19):1991-2002.
7. International Association of Diabetes and Pregnancy Study Groups Consensus Panel; Metzger BE, Gabbe SG, Persson B, Buchanan TA, Catalano PA, et al. International association of diabetes and pregnancy study groups recommendations on the diagnosis and classification of hyperglycemia in pregnancy. Diabetes Care. 2010;33(3):e98-82.
8. Government of India. Maternal and Health Division. National Guidelines for Diagnosis and Management of Gestational Diabetes Mellitus: Ministry of Health & Family Welfare. New Delhi, India: New Concept Information Systems; 2014.

7 CHAPTER

Management Options: Prevention and Treatment

INTRODUCTION

It is of utmost importance to maintain glycemic control during antenatal period. Various management options are available which are offered to patients in a stepwise manner including diet modifications, oral hypoglycemic drugs and insulin. In the following chapter indications and protocols for each management options have been described in detail.

PREVENTION

Lifestyle interventions (e.g., diet modification and exercise) are targeted at individuals at increased risk for developing gestational diabetes mellitus (GDM), particularly those who are overweight or obese and those with a history of GDM in a previous pregnancy.

Diet modification and increased exercise—in a meta-analysis of randomized trials, lifestyle interventions targeted at individuals with a higher baseline risk of GDM reduced the risk by approximately 20% compared with standard care. The interventions included diet modification, increased exercise, or both, ideally initiated before pregnancy and continuing across gestation; exercising at the proper intensity and frequency (e.g., moderate intensity for 50–60 minutes at least twice a week throughout pregnancy).

Individuals who are overweight or obese appear to benefit from weight loss before conception.

- Type of diet—The optimum diet is unclear. There is limited evidence that a diet favoring fruit, vegetables, whole grains, and fish and low in red and processed meat, refined grains, and high-fat dairy reduces the risk of developing GDM. The effect of a low glycemic index diet on risk of GDM is unclear as only a few small randomized trials have been performed.
- Smoking cessation—smoking cessation should be encouraged in all patients. Cessation has multiple maternal and fetal benefits and may reduce risk of GDM.

MEDICAL NUTRITION THERAPY

First line of management after the woman is diagnosed with gestational diabetes is diet and lifestyle modification. Medical nutrition therapy is individualized diet modification as per patient's lifestyle, weight, personal factors, and cultural practices. Upon diagnosis, patients with GDM should receive medical nutritional counseling by a registered dietitian (when possible) and be placed on an appropriate diet.

The goals of medical nutrition therapy is:

- To achieve normoglycemia
- To provide adequate nutrition
- To provide adequate gestational weight gain as per her body mass index (BMI)
- To provide adequate fetal well being.

Targets recommended by the Fifth International Workshop-Conference on GDM:[1]

- Fasting glucose <95 mg/dL (5.3 mmol/L) and either
- 1 hour postprandial glucose <140 mg/dL (7.8 mmol/L)
- 2 hours postprandial glucose <120 mg/dL (6.7 mmol/L).

Studies suggest that 70–85% of women diagnosed with GDM under Carpenter–Coustan criteria can control GDM with lifestyle modification alone. This proportion is anticipated to be even higher if the lower International Association of the Diabetes and Pregnancy Study Groups[2] diagnostic thresholds are used.

The total calorie intake varies according to the BMI of the woman.[3]

- BMI <25 kg/m^2—3,000 cal/day
- Overweight (BMI 25–30 kg/m^2)—2,500 cal/day
- Morbid obesity (BMI 40 kg/m^2)—1,250 cal/day

The total calorie requirement should consist of, 45% carbohydrate, 30% protein, and 25% fat (mainly unsaturated fats). The caloric requirement of the patient should be met by three major meals and three small meals at equal intervals.[3]

Carbohydrate intake: In a meta-analysis of randomized trials of dietary intervention in patients with GDM, low carbohydrate diets had a favorable effect on postprandial blood glucose concentrations and significantly lowered the need for insulin therapy but did not affect other maternal or newborn outcomes. Increasing fiber intake preferably through food (vegetables, fruits, legumes, and intact whole grains) may help to modestly lower A1C and at the same time promote eating lower glycemic index foods.[4] We usually limit carbohydrate intake to 40% of the meal while preventing ketonuria. Many women will require individualized adjustments of carbohydrates by 15–30 g in each meal to lower postprandial glucose levels which are directly related to carbohydrate content.

Protein intake: Remaining calorie requirement of 20–30% is gained from proteins. Protein intake should be evenly distributed throughout the day with three major and minor meals to improve satiety, slow carbohydrate absorption, and provide calories. High protein snack at bedtime prevents overnight starvation and ketosis and maintains fasting glucose levels.

Fat intake: 25% of total calorie intake with majority being unsaturated fatty acids.

It is important to pay attention to subsequent changes in weight following dietary modifications. In a retrospective cohort study including over 31,000 patients with GDM, those with appropriate gestational weight gain had optimal outcomes, while excessive gestational weight gain was associated with a significantly increased risk of having a large for gestational age newborn, preterm birth, and caesarean birth.[5]

Exercise: Women with gestational diabetes are encouraged to perform 30–60 minutes of moderate-intensity aerobic exercises like brisk walking, cycling, or swimming on most days of the week (at least 150 minutes a week). Exercise that increases muscle mass, including aerobic, resistance, and circuit training, appears to improve glucose management, primarily from increased tissue sensitivity to insulin. As a result, both fasting and postprandial glucose levels are controlled and the need for pharmacological therapy is obviated.

PHARMACOTHERAPY

The goal of pharmacotherapy is to manage glucose levels so that the majority are no higher than the upper limit of the target range, without inducing any episodes of hypoglycemia.

Indications of Pharmacotherapy

- Blood glucose targets not reached by medical nutrition therapy.
- To prevent fetal macrosomia. Data from some randomized trials suggest that pharmacotherapy in the form of insulin or oral hypoglycemic drugs can reduce occurrence of macrosomia and large for gestational age births.

Oral hypoglycemic drugs: Two oral hypoglycemic agents (OHAs) have been used in pregnancy—metformin (biguanide group) and glyburide (sulphonylurea group). In the past, there was concern regarding the teratogenecity of these drugs due to their transplacental transfer. Although insulin is considered the first line of management for gestational diabetes, both American College of Obstetricians and Gynecologists (2017a) and the ADA (2017b) acknowledge that several studies support the safety and efficacy of either glyburide (micronase) or metformin (glucophage).

Metformin: The Metformin in Gestational diabetes (MIG) trial showed that use of metformin in GDM patients reduced the required dose of insulin and also reduced the total weight gain.[6] There was, however, no difference in the perinatal outcome. Patient acceptability was better. Typical dose of metformin starts with 500 mg extended release once a day. The dose can then be increased by 500–1,000 mg orally per week until reaching the usual effective dose of 1,500–2,000 mg orally per day divided into two doses (maximum daily dose is 2,500 mg).[6] Side effects of metformin are gastrointestinal, including a metallic taste in the mouth, mild anorexia, nausea, abdominal discomfort, and diarrhea. These symptoms are usually mild, transient, and reversible after dose reduction or discontinuation of the drug. Symptoms can be avoided by starting at a low dose with slow-dose escalation. Metformin reaches fetal serum concentrations similar to maternal levels. Short-term perinatal outcomes between insulin and metformin did not differ. Outcomes included neonatal hypoglycemia, respiratory distress syndrome, phototherapy, birth trauma, 5-minute Apgar score ≤7, and preterm birth. Overall growth of offspring at age 2 years also did not differ.

Glyburide: Although evidence suggests that glyburide in the dose of 5–10 mg BD appears to be safe for the fetus, it did not have any added advantage over insulin in treatment of GDM.[7] Like metformin, glyburide also crosses the placenta and reaches concentrations in the fetus that are more than two-thirds of maternal levels. A significant rise in rates of neonatal intensive care unit admission, respiratory distress, and neonatal hypoglycemia was associated with glyburide use. Most common side effect of glyburide was maternal hypoglycemia.

Choosing metformin versus glyburide—Clinically important pregnancy outcomes are generally similar for metformin and glyburide, with only limited evidence of benefit of one oral medication over the other.

Pregnancy outcome—When compared with glyburide in meta-analyses of randomized trials, metformin resulted in:

- Similar rates of perinatal mortality, neonatal hypoglycemia,[8] and hypertensive disorders of pregnancy[9]
- Lower mean birth weight[10]
- Less macrosomia and large for gestational age[10]
- Less gestational weight gain[10]

Need for supplemental insulin that is failure rate of metformin and glyburide are similar. If oral pharmacotherapy alone does not adequately manage glucose levels, supplemental insulin can be prescribed and may be easier for the patient than switching to a multi-dose insulin only regimen. In contrast to nonpregnant patients, dual use of oral agents (e.g., metformin plus glyburide) is not recommended in pregnancy because of minimal safety and efficacy data and concerns about adverse fetal effects since both drugs cross the placenta.

Insulin: Insulin is typically considered as the gold standard first line of management for gestational diabetes. It does not cross placenta and helps in tight control of blood glucose levels. Insulin is started when medical nutrition therapy alone does not meet glucose targets. Traditionally, short-acting regular insulin is recommended (onset of action 30 minutes lasting for 6–8 hours) and intermediate-acting neutral protamine Hagedorn (NPH) insulin (onset of action 1 hour, lasting for 10–14 hours). Recent research has added newer rapid-acting insulin lispro and aspart whose action begins within 15 minutes. A study on glargine (long-acting insulin) observed no increased adverse outcome compared to NPH. However, glargine has still not been recommended for use in pregnancy due to concerns regarding its mitogenic action and causing increased fetal growth due to high affinity for the insulin-like growth factor receptor-1.[11]

Dose of insulin: Insulin requirement increases with increase in gestational age, glycemic control, obesity, and other factors. If insulin is initiated, the starting dose is typically 0.7 units/kg/day to 2 units/kg/day and is given in divided doses (American College of Obstetricians and Gynecologists, 2017a). As per gestational age, 0.9 units/kg is given in second trimester and 1 unit/kg is given in second trimester. Adjustment to the above regimen is needed in case of obesity. Dose titration to blood glucose levels is based upon frequent monitoring. At least four daily glucose measurements are required (fasting and 1 or 2 hours postprandial with the addition of prelunch and predinner measurements as needed) to optimize therapy and ensure timely dose increases. Since any insulin regimen requires serial dosing adjustments in response to specific fasting or postprandial glucose levels, the starting dose should be considered just that, a starting point. The patient's glucose log should be reviewed weekly so that insulin doses can be adjusted as needed to meet target glucose levels as the pregnancy advances.

Commonly used formula for insulin therapy is:

$$\text{Total daily insulin requirement} = 2/3 \text{ in the morning} + 1/3 \text{ at night}$$

$$\text{Such that morning dose} = 2/3 \text{ NPH} + 1/3 \text{ short-acting}$$

$$\text{Predinner dose} = 1/2 \text{ NPH} + 1/2 \text{ short-acting}$$

Hospitalization is not routine for starting insulin therapy unless teaching patients to administer insulin is not possible on outpatient basis.

Following points are given as an alternative pragmatic approach for adjusting insulin as per glucose monitoring.

- We begin with a single injection of 10–20 units of intermediate-acting basal insulin (NPH) and 6–10 units of rapid-acting insulin (lispro or aspart) in the morning immediately before breakfast; the dose within this range is based on the degree of elevation above target levels.

- If postprandial glucose levels throughout the day remain high, adjustments in the rapid-acting insulin dose are typically in the range of 10–20%.
- If only the postdinner glucose level remains elevated, then we add an injection of 6–10 units of rapid-acting insulin immediately before dinner.
- If only the postlunch glucose level remains elevated, we add an injection of 6–10 units of rapid-acting insulin immediately before lunch. If both postbreakfast and postlunch glucose levels are elevated, increasing the morning NPH may be sufficient.
- If the fasting glucose level is elevated after postprandial levels in the target range, we add an intermediate-acting basal insulin, preferably at bedtime but with dinner is another option on an individualized basis.

Intermittent home blood glucose monitoring: Patients should monitor their own glucose levels. All available glucose meters measure plasma equivalent of capillary blood glucose. It is recommended that patients should monitor their blood glucose at least once before breakfast (fasting) and at 1 or 2 hours postprandial after both lunch and dinner.[12,13] Checking preprandial levels have shown to be of lesser benefit as compared to postprandial. Postprandial values also help in better adjusting short-acting insulin. Reducing blood glucose monitoring to every alternate day in well-controlled patients on medical nutrition therapy alone or pharmacotherapy (glucose levels 5–10 mg/dL above targets, no evidence of fetal macrosomia with effective fetal weight <90th centile, normal amniotic fluid) does not increase the incidence of adverse outcomes but improves patient's quality of life. Although use of CGM has no clear advantages for most patients based on available data, it may be considered on an individualized basis in patients who cannot consistently check finger stick glucose levels and are willing to wear a device.

REFERENCES

1. Metzger BE, Buchanan TA, Coustan DR, de Leiva A, Dunger DB, Hadden DR, et al. Summary and recommendations of the Fifth International Workshop-Conference on Gestational Diabetes Mellitus. Diabetes Care. 2007;30 (Supplement_2):S251-60.
2. Mayo K, Melamed N, Vandenberghe H, Berger H. The impact of adoption of the International Association of Diabetes in Pregnancy Study Group criteria for the screening and diagnosis of gestational diabetes. Am J Obstet Gynecol. 2015;212(2):224.e1-9.
3. Duarte-Gardea MO, Gonzales-Pacheco DM, Reader DM, Thomas AM, Wang SR, Gregory RP, et al. Academy of Nutrition and Dietetics Gestational Diabetes Evidence-Based Nutrition Practice Guideline. J Acad Nutr Diet. 2018;118(9):1719-42.
4. Evert AB, Dennison M, Gardner CD, Garvey WT, Lau KHK, MacLeod J, et al. Nutrition therapy for adults with diabetes or prediabetes: A consensus report. Diabetes Care. 2019;42(5):731-54.

5. Cheng YW, Chung JH, Kurbisch-Block I, Inturrisi M, Shafer S, Caughey AB. Gestational weight gain and gestational diabetes mellitus: perinatal outcomes. Obstet Gynecol. 2008;112(5):1015-22.
6. Rowan JA, Hague WM, Gao W, Battin MR, Moore MP; MiG Trial Investigators. Metformin versus insulin for the treatment of gestational diabetes. N Engl J Med. 2008;358(19):2003-15.
7. Hebert MF, Ma X, Naraharisetti SB, Krudys KM, Umans JG, Hankins GD, et al. Are we optimizing gestational diabetes treatment with glyburide? The pharmacologic basis for better clinical practice. Clin Pharmacol Ther. 2009; 85:607-14.
8. Brown J, Martis R, Hughes B, Rowan J, Crowther CA. Oral anti-diabetic pharmacological therapies for the treatment of women with gestational diabetes. Cochrane Database Syst Rev. 2017;1(1):CD011967.
9. Kalafat E, Sukur YE, Abdi A, Thilaganathan B, Khalil A. Metformin for prevention of hypertensive disorders of pregnancy in women with gestational diabetes or obesity: systematic review and meta-analysis of randomized trials. Ultrasound Obstet Gynecol. 2018;52(6):706-14.
10. Tarry-Adkins JL, Aiken CE, Ozanne SE. Comparative impact of pharmacological treatments for gestational diabetes on neonatal anthropometry independent of maternal glycaemic control: A systematic review and meta-analysis. PLoS Med. 2020;17(5):e1003126.
11. Pollex E, Morreti ME, Koren G, Feig D. Safety of insulin glargine use in pregnancy: A systematic review and meta-analysis. Ann Pharmacother. 2011;45(1):9-16.
12. Laird J, McFarland KF. Fasting blood glucose levels and initiation of insulin therapy in gestational diabetes. Endocr Pract. 1996;2(5):330-2.
13. Moses RG, Lucas EM, Knights S. Gestational diabetes mellitus. At what time should the postprandial glucose level be monitored? Aust N Z J Obstet Gynaecol. 1999;39(4):457-60.

8 CHAPTER

Labor Management and Intrapartum Fetal Surveillance

INTRODUCTION

Diabetes during pregnancy whether pregestational or gestational, poses unique challenges, including an increased risk of maternal and neonatal complications. These may include macrosomia, shoulder dystocia, preterm labor and neonatal hypoglycemia, necessitating careful planning and monitoring during labor and delivery. Key considerations include glycemic control, timing of delivery and mode of delivery.

TIMING OF DELIVERY

One of the key issues with gestational diabetes is the timing of delivery. The optimal timing of birth in gestational diabetes mellitus (GDM) has not been evaluated in well-designed trials and the available data is inadequate to allow a strong evidence-based recommendation.[1] The potential benefits of early induction of labor is preventing late still birth and avoiding complications related to macrosomia, i.e., shoulder dystocia and increased rates of caesarean section.[2] The disadvantages of early induction are risks of induction and increased neonatal morbidity and neonatal intensive care unit (ICU) admission. Although most associations recommend delivery after 38 completed weeks of gestation in a diabetic patient, some state that uncomplicated cases of gestational diabetes (not pregestational) may be allowed to wait for spontaneous labor up to 40 weeks with adequate fetal surveillance. Some institutions follow glycemic control as an indicator for timing of delivery. This is based on whether the patient is A1 or A2 GDM with adequate glycemic control.

A1 GDM with good glycemic control: These are patients that remain euglycemic throughout pregnancy with medical nutrition therapy and exercise alone. General consensus is that such patients should not be induced before 39^{+0} weeks of gestation and after 41^{+0} weeks of gestation. This relatively noninterventional approach is based on the favorable outcomes reported in a classic uncontrolled case series of 196 patients with class A diabetes managed this way.[3]

A2 GDM or A1 GDM with poor glycemic control: Patients on pharmacotherapy such oral hypoglycemic agents or insulin are considered as A2 GDM. The American College of Obstetricians and Gynecologists (ACOG) suggests patient with A2 GDM with good glycemic control should be induced between 39^{+0} and 39^{+6} weeks of gestation. Patients with A1 GDM with suboptimal glucose control, it is suggested to induce at 39^{+0} weeks of gestation based on data from a retrospective cohort study of patients with GDM suggesting that the infant mortality rate at 39^{+0} weeks was statistically lower than the risk of stillbirth plus infant mortality with expectant management over an additional week.[4]

Guidance for patients with suboptimal glycemic control on pharmacologic therapy is less precise. They suggest birth at 37^{+0}–38^{+6} weeks of gestation may be reasonable, but that birth prior to 37^{+0} weeks should only be initiated when more aggressive efforts to control blood glucose levels, such as hospitalization, have failed.[5]

Mode of delivery: The ACOG and National Institute for Health and Care Excellence guidelines suggest that vaginal delivery is not contraindicated for suspected macrosomia unless the estimated fetal weight is 4.5 kg. In the Indian population, the average baby weight is less. Balaji et al. in their study on the diagnosis of GDM in Indian women considered birth weight of 90th centile, which is 3.45 kg, as macrosomia.[6] Vaginal delivery can be offered after thorough pelvic assessment and induction of labor can be done by mechanical method or prostaglandins.

Labor analgesia can be offered.

For women with diabetes and comorbidities such as obesity or autonomic neuropathy, offer an anesthetic assessment in the third trimester of pregnancy.[7]

If the woman has general anesthesia for the birth, monitor blood glucose every 30 minutes from induction of general anesthesia until after the baby is born and the woman is fully conscious.[7]

Glycemic monitoring during labor and birth—insulin requirements usually decrease during labor as oral caloric intake is reduced and the work of labor, particularly uterine contractions, requires extra energy. Hyperglycemia is treated to prevent neonatal hypoglycemia. Aim is to keep glucose level between 72 and 126 mg/dL.

A1 GDM—patients with GDM who were euglycemic without use of insulin or oral antihyperglycemic medications during pregnancy generally do not develop hyperglycemia during labor and birth and thus do not need their blood glucose levels checked. However some institutes prefer to monitor blood glucose levels of such patients due to concerns about the validity of outpatient self-monitored glycemic assessments. Patients undergoing elective caesarean section with A1 GDM which is well controlled have management similar to normal antenatal patients.

A2 GDM—patients on pharmacotherapy for GDM may require insulin during labor to maintain blood glucose in the target range.

On the evening prior to induction (if indicated), insulin dose and meal are taken by the patient. Morning dose of insulin is omitted and fasting blood glucose done.

Subcutaneous correctional insulin—patients with gestational diabetes can often be managed with subcutaneous correctional insulin during labor (refer to following text). If blood glucose levels >125 mg/dL despite subcutaneous insulin, insulin infusion can be initiated.

Two intravenous (IV) lines must be secured. If blood glucose level is not maintained then dextrose insulin neutralizing drip is started. 50 units of regular insulin in 500 mL of normal saline is started. Dose is adjusted according to glucose level:

- 90 mg/dL—0.5 U/h
- 90–126 mg/dL–1U/h
- 126–180 mg/dL–2U/h
- 180–240 mg/dL–3U/h
- 240 mg/dL–4U/h

10% dextrose drip at the rate of 125 mL/h is continuously given through the other line. It is important to monitor vitals and fluid intake and output, urinary ketones, and blood glucose level 1–2 hourly. Fetal heart must be continuously monitored and partograph be charted in active labor.

Patients for elective caesarean section: They should be scheduled early in the morning. Patients on multiple daily injections should maintain their usual dose of neutral protaminehagedorn (NPH) on the night prior to admission. If they use a longer-acting basal insulin at night, the dose should be decreased by 20–50%, with the exact percentage dose reduction determined by the risk of morning hypoglycemia. Morning dose of insulin should be skipped and if the caesarean will be delayed past the early morning, 50–70% of the usual basal insulin dose can be given and intravenous dextrose should be administered if the blood glucose is below 100 mg/dL. Pre- and intraoperative hyperglycemia is treated with either intravenous insulin or subcutaneous rapid-acting insulin, as needed, to manage glucose levels. Patients on metformin should skip the morning dose of metformin.

Precautions during caesarean: Elective caesarean for macrosomia is recommended in a diabetic pregnancy if the estimated fetal weight is 4.5 kg (ACOG). Anesthetist must be consulted prior to elective surgery. Special precautions while performing the section are adequate incision size to allow delivery of the big baby, use of forceps to deliver high floating head, to check for and suture extensions of the uterine incision which may take place especially while performing a second stage caesarean. Postoperative glucose monitoring must be continued and patient must be mobilized as early as possible.

INDUCTION OF LABOR

Patients undergoing induction of labor can be managed similarly to those who have spontaneous labor. In patients on long-acting basal insulin (>24 hours duration of action), particularly multiparous patients who may have a shorter labor, some clinicians reduce the dose by 20–50% on the night prior to an induction of labor.

Continuous electronic fetal monitoring is recommended for patients with GDM in labor.

REFERENCES

1. Feghali MN, Caritis SN, Catov JM, Scifres CM. Timing of delivery and pregnancy outcomes in women with gestational diabetes. Am J Obstet Gynecol. 2016;215(2):243.e1-7.
2. Lurie S, Insler V, Hagay ZJ. Induction of labor at 38 to 39 weeks of gestation reduces the incidence of shoulder dystocia in gestational diabetic patients class A2. Am J Perinatol. 1996;13(5):293-6.
3. Gabbe SG, Mestman JG, Freeman RK, Anderson GV, Lowensohn RI. Management and outcome of class A diabetes mellitus. Am J Obstet Gynecol. 1977;127(5):465-9.
4. Rosenstein MG, Cheng YW, Snowden JM, Nicholson JM, Doss AE, Caughey AB. The risk of stillbirth and infant death stratified by gestational age in women with gestational diabetes. Am J Obstet Gynecol. 2012;206(4):309.e1-7.
5. ACOG Practice Bulletin No. 190: Gestational Diabetes Mellitus. Obstet Gynecol. 2018;131(2):e49-e64.
6. Balaji V, Balaji M, Anjalakshi C, Cynthia A, Arthi T, Seshiah V. Diagnosis of gestational diabetes in Asian-Indian women. Indian J Endocr Metab. 2011;15(3):187-90.
7. NICE guideline. (2015). Diabetes in pregnancy: management from preconception to the postnatal period. [online] Available from https://www.nice.org.uk/guidance/ng3/resources/diabetes-in-pregnancy-management-from-preconception-to-the-postnatal-period-51038446021 [Last accessed November, 2024].

9 CHAPTER Postpartum Care

CARE OF DIABETIC INFANT

INTRODUCTION

Diabetes in pregnancy is associated with an increased risk of fetal, neonatal, and long-term complications in the offspring. The risk of complications in the offspring varies considerably depending upon whether the mother has pregestational or gestational diabetes mellitus (PGDM or GDM), whether the mother is insulin-dependent, and the degree of glycemic control achieved before and during pregnancy. Refer to **Table 1** for the list of complications.[1]

DELIVERY ROOM CARE

Neonatal resuscitation should be assessed properly based on the gestational age, predicted birth weight, prenatally diagnosed congenital anomalies, mode of delivery, and any complications of labor including any birth injuries.

TABLE 1: Fetal complications of gestational diabetes mellitus.

Congenital abnormalities	*Neonatal complications*
• Congenital heart disease: – Transposition of great arteries – Ventricular septal defects – Atrial septal defects – Patent ductus arteriosus – Tricuspid atresia – Truncus arteriosus – Double outlet right ventricle – Coarctation of aorta – Hypoplastic left heart syndrome and other single outlet syndromes • Neural tube defects: – Anencephaly – Spina bifida • Caudal regression syndrome • Small left colon syndrome • Cleft palate • Vertebral anomalies • Flexion contracture of limbs • Intestinal anomalies	• Prematurity • Macrosomia/large for gestational age (LGA) babies: – Including all birth related complications and injuries • Perinatal hypoxia • Respiratory distress syndrome • Metabolic complications: – Hypoglycemia – Hypocalcemia – Hypomagnesemia – Cardiomyopathy • Haematological complications: – Low iron stores – Polycythemia • Hyperbilirubinemia

A trained team should attend and provide care specifically to the infant. The initial evaluation determines the need for further interventions. The infant should have timely skin-to-skin care and initiation of breastfeeding in the delivery room.

Infants of diabetic mothers are at increased risk of metabolic disturbances in the newborn period especially hypoglycemia, hypocalcemia, and hypomagnesemia.

HYPOGLYCEMIA

The onset of hypoglycemia typically occurs within the first few hours after birth. Thus, these infants require close blood glucose monitoring after delivery and frequently need enteral or parenteral glucose supplementation. Large for gestational age (LGA) infants are likely to develop hypoglycemia as well as small for gestational age (SGA) as their glycogen stores are reduced, and hyperinsulinemia impairs the ability to mobilize hepatic glycogen.[2,3] Hypoglycemia is caused by persistent hyperinsulinemia in the newborn after intrauterine glucose supply from the mother has stopped.

HYPOCALCEMIA

Hypocalcemia occurs in approximately 5% of diabetic infants, though some studies have reported rates as high as 30%.[4,5] Hypocalcemia is mostly asymptomatic and resolves without treatment. As a result, routine screening is not necessary. However, calcium levels should be measured in infants with signs of hypocalcemia (jitteriness, lethargy, apnea, tachypnea, or seizures, and in those with prematurity, asphyxia, and respiratory distress).

HYPOMAGNESEMIA

Hypomagnesemia occurs in up to 40% of infants of mothers with diabetes (IMD) within the first 3 days after birth. It is usually transient and asymptomatic, hence does not require screening or treatment. Hypomagnesemia, however can sometimes reduce both parathyroid hormone secretion and responsiveness. Hence, some babies with both hypocalcemia and hypomagnesemia may not respond to calcium alone.[6,7]

Polycythemia, defined as a central venous hematocrit of >65%, is more likely in IMD compared with infants whose mothers are not diabetic.[1] Polycythemia may lead to hyperviscosity syndrome, including vascular sludging, ischemia, and infarction of vital organs.

Hyperbilirubinemia occurs in 10–30% of infants of mothers with diabetes. The risk is particularly high in preterm neonates.

RESPIRATORY DISTRESS SYNDROME

At a given gestational age, infants of diabetic mother are more likely to develop respiratory distress syndrome (RDS) because maternal hyperglycemia appears to impair or delay surfactant synthesis. The proposed underlying mechanism is neonatal hyperinsulinemia, which interferes with the induction of lung maturation by glucocorticoids.[8]

Macrosomia or LGA [defined as birth weight (BW) >4,000 g or >90th percentile for gestational age], is a common complication of diabetic pregnancies. The incidence is greatest in infants born to mothers with pregestational diabetes mellitus.[9] Infants with macrosomia are more likely than those who are not macrosomic to have hyperbilirubinemia, hypoglycemia, acidosis, respiratory distress, shoulder dystocia, and brachial plexus injury.

BREASTFEEDING, CONTRACEPTION, POSTPARTUM FOLLOW-UP

POSTPARTUM FOLLOW-UP

Patients with gestational diabetes should resume a normal diet postpartum.

BREASTFEEDING

Breastfeeding is encouraged postpartum in patients of gestational diabetes as it is beneficial for both the baby and the mother. Breastfeeding has shown to improve glucose metabolism and reduce glucose levels obtained during a postpartum glucose tolerance test.[10] Several prospective studies have reported that breastfeeding decreased the long-term incidence of type 2 diabetes after a diagnosis of GDM compared with not breastfeeding.

CONTRACEPTION

All contraception are acceptable as long as there no medical contraindications to their use. There is no convincing evidence that hormonal contraceptives (estrogen-progestin or progestin-only) increase the user's risk of developing type 1 or type 2 diabetes.[11] If there is still concern then copper intrauterine contraceptive device (IUCD) is a good alternative.

SCREENING FOR OVERT DIABETES

The hyperglycemic effect of placental hormones quickly dissipates postdelivery and patients revert back to their glycemic status before pregnancy, ranging from immediately to within a week. Most patients do not require hypoglycemic medications postdelivery.

Since some patients with GDM may have previously unrecognized type 2 diabetes mellitus, we check glucose concentrations postpartum to exclude ongoing hyperglycemia. In a patient with A1 GDM, it is common to check only a single fasting glucose and, if normal, stop checking blood glucose values. In a patient with A2 GDM, we usually check glucose levels for 24 hours, obtaining both fasting and postprandial blood glucose values and if normal stop checking them. However, if any values are abnormal then they are treated medically as overt diabetes.

Patients with normal/near normal postpartum should undergo a 2-hour 75-g oral glucose tolerance test 4–12 weeks after delivery. If levels are abnormal, they are to be treated medically as overt diabetes, and the risks for future complications are to be explained.

REFERENCES

1. Riskin A, Itzchaki O, Bader D, Iofe A, Toropine A, Riskin-Mashiah S. Perinatal Outcomes in Infants of Mothers with Diabetes in Pregnancy. Isr Med Assoc J. 2020;22(9):569-75.
2. Metzger BE, Persson B, Lowe LP, Dyer AR, Cruickshank JK, Deerochanawong C, et al.; HAPO Study Cooperative Research Group. Hyperglycemia and adverse pregnancy outcome study: neonatal glycemia. Pediatrics. 2010;126(6):e1545-52.
3. Kalhan SC, Savin SM, Adam PA. Attenuated glucose production rate in newborn infants of insulin-dependent diabetic mothers. N Engl J Med. 1977;296(7):375-6.
4. Cordero L, Treuer SH, Landon MB, Gabbe SG. Management of infants of diabetic mothers. Arch Pediatr Adolesc Med. 1998;152(3):249-54.
5. Demarini S, Mimouni F, Tsang RC, Khoury J, Hertzberg V. Impact of metabolic control of diabetes during pregnancy on neonatal hypocalcemia: a randomized study. Obstet Gynecol. 1994;83(6):918-22.
6. Tsang RC, Strub R, Brown DR, Steichen J, Hartman C, Chen IW. Hypomagnesemia in infants of diabetic mothers: perinatal studies. J Pediatr. 1976;89(1):115-9.
7. Banerjee S, Mimouni FB, Mehta R, Llanos A, Bainbridge R, Varada K, et al. Lower whole blood ionized magnesium concentrations in hypocalcemic infants of gestational diabetic mothers. Magnes Res. 2003;16(2):127-30.
8. Bourbon JR, Farrell PM. Fetal lung development in the diabetic pregnancy. Pediatr Res. 1985;19(3):253-67.
9. Kong L, Nilsson IAK, Gissler M, Lavebratt C. Associations of maternal diabetes and body mass index with offspring birth weight and prematurity. JAMA Pediatr. 2019;173(4):371-8.
10. Lenz S, Kühl C, Hornnes PJ, Hagen C. Influence of lactation on oral glucose tolerance in the puerperium. Acta Endocrinol (Copenh). 1981;98(3):428-31.
11. Lopez LM, Grimes DA, Schulz KF. Steroidal contraceptives: effect on carbohydrate metabolism in women without diabetes mellitus. Cochrane Database Syst Rev. 2014;2014(4):CD006133. Update in: Cochrane Database Syst Rev. 2019;2019(11).

10

CHAPTER

Long-term Consequences to the Offspring

INTRODUCTION

The intrauterine environment plays a crucial role in shaping and infants growth and metabolism. In pregnancies complicated by diabetes, especially when poorly controlled, the fetus is exposed to hyperglycemia, leading to developmental programming that may predispose the child to chronic conditions later in life.

DIABETES

Maternal diabetic intrauterine environment is strongly associated with type 2 diabetes mellitus (T2DM) development in the offspring.[1] The offspring of mothers with gestational diabetes mellitus (GDM) history have at least 5 times greater risk of developing impaired glucose tolerance than those not exposed to gestational diabetes. More than two-thirds of offspring of mothers with gestational diabetes developed T2DM by 34 years of age.[2]

OBESITY

Fetal hyperinsulinemia, caused by intrauterine exposure to hyperglycemia, may affect the development of adipose tissue and pancreatic beta cells leading to impaired glucose metabolism and increased risk for obesity in later childhood and adulthood. This can occur both in offspring of mother with pregestational and gestational diabetes.[3,4]

ENDOCRINE MORBIDITY

The GDM leads to the risk of long-term endocrine morbidity in the offspring. The incidence of diabetes mellitus, overweight, and obesity among children was significantly higher in the GDM group. The rates of hypothyroidism were comparable between the groups.

CARDIOVASCULAR MORBIDITY

A significant association was recently noted between GDM and the rate of cardiovascular hospitalizations of the offspring.[5]

NEURODEVELOPMENTAL OUTCOME

Though poor maternal glycemic control can adversely affect the developing brain,[6] it is important to note that neurodevelopmental outcomes of infants of mothers with well-controlled diabetes are similar to those of infants of nondiabetic mothers.[7] Increasing HbA1C levels are associated with decreasing head circumference and decreased intellectual performance at 3 years of age. Elevated maternal ketone concentrations during the second and third trimesters decrease psychomotor development at 6–9 years.

REFERENCES

1. Reece EA, Homko CJ. Infant of the diabetic mother. Semin Perinatol. 1994;18(5):459-69.
2. Dabelea D, Knowler WC, Pettitt DJ. Effect of diabetes in pregnancy on offspring: follow-up research in the Pima Indians. J Matern Fetal Med. 2000;9(1): 83-8.
3. Mughal MZ, Eelloo J, Roberts SA, Maresh M, Ward KA, Ashby R, et al. Body composition and bone status of children born to mothers with type 1 diabetes mellitus. Arch Dis Child. 2010;95(4):281-5.
4. Page KA, Romero A, Buchanan TA, Xiang AH. Gestational diabetes mellitus, maternal obesity, and adiposity in offspring. J Pediatr. 2014;164(4):807-10.
5. Leybovitz-Haleluya N, Wainstock T, Landau D, Sheiner E. Maternal gestational diabetes mellitus and the risk of subsequent pediatric cardiovascular diseases of the offspring: a population-based cohort study with up to 18 years of follow up. Acta Diabetol. 2018;55:1037-42.
6. Adane AA, Mishra GD, Tooth LR. Diabetes in pregnancy and childhood cognitive development: A systematic review. Pediatrics. 2016;137(5):e20154234.
7. Boghossian NS, Hansen NI, Bell EF, Brumbaugh JE, Stoll BJ, Laptook AR, et al. Eunice Kennedy Shriver National Institute of Child Health and Human Development Neonatal Research Network. Outcomes of extremely preterm infants born to insulin-dependent diabetic mothers. Pediatrics. 2016;137(6):e20153424.

CHAPTER 11

Multiple Choice Questions

1. **What is gestational diabetes?**
   a. A form of diabetes that occurs after childbirth
   b. A form of diabetes that occurs during pregnancy
   c. A form of diabetes that occurs in childhood
   d. A form of diabetes that occurs in elderly individuals

Ans. b. A form of diabetes that occurs during pregnancy

2. **What is the most common time for gestational diabetes to be diagnosed?**
   a. Before pregnancy
   b. First trimester
   c. Second trimester
   d. Third trimester

Ans. c. Second trimester

3. **Which of the following is NOT a risk factor for gestational diabetes?**
   a. Obesity
   b. Family history of diabetes
   c. Being younger than 25 years old
   d. Previous pregnancy with gestational diabetes

Ans. c. Being younger than 25 years old

4. **What is the primary concern for the baby if the mother has gestational diabetes?**
   a. Low birth weight
   b. High birth weight (macrosomia)
   c. Premature delivery
   d. Neural tube defects

Ans. b. High birth weight (macrosomia)

5. **Which of the following tests is commonly used to diagnose gestational diabetes?**
   a. Oral glucose tolerance test (OGTT)
   b. Fasting blood glucose test
   c. HbA1c test
   d. Insulin sensitivity test

Ans. a. Oral glucose tolerance test (OGTT)

6. Which of the following complications is associated with untreated gestational diabetes?

a. Low blood pressure in the mother
b. Preeclampsia
c. Thyroid dysfunction
d. Vitamin D deficiency

Ans. b. Preeclampsia

7. Women with gestational diabetes are at increased risk of developing which condition later in life?

a. Type 1 diabetes
b. Type 2 diabetes
c. Hypoglycemia
d. Celiac disease

Ans. b. Type 2 diabetes

8. What is the typical recommendation for women with gestational diabetes after delivery?

a. Continue diabetes medications
b. No further monitoring is required
c. Undergo regular blood glucose monitoring
d. Immediate insulin therapy

Ans. c. Undergo regular blood glucose monitoring

9. Which hormone plays a major role in the development of gestational diabetes by causing insulin resistance?

a. Estrogen
b. Progesterone
c. Human placental lactogen (hPL)
d. Cortisol

Ans. c. Human placental lactogen (hPL)

10. What is the first-line approach in managing gestational diabetes during pregnancy?

a. Oral medications like metformin
b. Insulin injections
c. Diet and lifestyle modifications
d. Immediate induction of labor

Ans. c. Diet and lifestyle modifications

11. Which of the following blood glucose levels is considered the target fasting blood glucose for women with gestational diabetes?

a. Less than 120 mg/dL
b. 70–95 mg/dL
c. 100–130 mg/dL
d. Less than 150 mg/dL

Ans. b. 70–95 mg/dL

12. When should insulin therapy be initiated in women with gestational diabetes?
 a. If diet and exercise fail to control blood glucose levels
 b. As soon as gestational diabetes is diagnosed
 c. Only during labor
 d. Insulin is not recommended for GDM management

Ans. a. If diet and exercise fail to control blood glucose levels

13. What is the preferred method of delivery for women with well-controlled gestational diabetes?
 a. Caesarean section
 b. Induced labor at 36 weeks
 c. Spontaneous vaginal delivery at term
 d. Elective caesarean at 37 weeks

Ans. c. Spontaneous vaginal delivery at term

14. What is the main goal in managing gestational diabetes during labor?
 a. Preventing neonatal hypoglycemia
 b. Avoiding premature labor
 c. Reducing maternal weight gain
 d. Preventing maternal hypotension

Ans. a. Preventing neonatal hypoglycemia

15. What is the recommended blood glucose target for a woman with GDM during labor?
 a. Less than 180 mg/dL
 b. 90–110 mg/dL
 c. 120–150 mg/dL
 d. 140–160 mg/dL

Ans. b. 90–110 mg/dL

16. What is the appropriate management of insulin during labor in women with gestational diabetes?
 a. Stop insulin therapy immediately upon admission
 b. Continue prepregnancy insulin doses
 c. Administer a continuous insulin infusion to maintain target glucose levels
 d. Avoid insulin and focus on hydration

Ans. c. Administer a continuous insulin infusion to maintain target glucose levels

17. When is postpartum glucose testing recommended for women who had gestational diabetes?
 a. 1 week after delivery
 b. 6 weeks postpartum
 c. 3 months postpartum
 d. No postpartum glucose testing is required

Ans. b. 6 weeks postpartum

Index

Page numbers followed by *f* refer to figure, *fc* refer to flowchart, and *t* refer to table.